DEDICATION

This book is dedicated to my trainer, Coach Francis. You helped transform a nerd to the man every guy wants to be. Thank you.

Table of Contents

CHAPTER 1- WHY BODY BUILDING IS OFTEN MISUNDERSTOOD

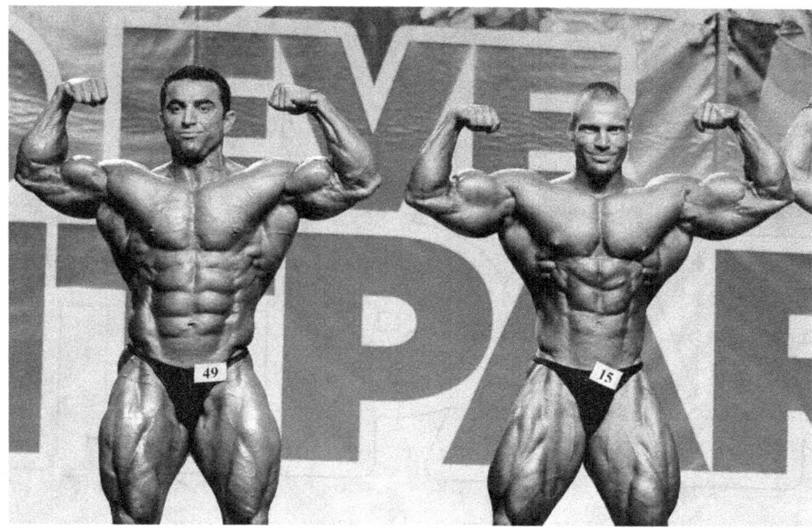

Many people misunderstand the purpose of or principle behind bodybuilding. It's much more than just to gain huge muscles and become extremely strong. Any time we want to improve a part of our body such as to become slimmer, have better curves or just improve our overall shape, we need to perform certain bodybuilding activities.

However, often bodybuilding by itself may not be enough; we may also need to enroll in some sort of slimming or diet program. Learning the basic principles of bodybuilding can help you to get on the right bodybuilding program and achieve the body of your dreams.

What's Your Current Body Size and Weight?

Before you begin your bodybuilding, take measurements of all your body parts including waist, chest, hips, forearms, upper arms, calves, thighs, etc. Knowing what your beginning measurements are is the best way to monitor your progress. Just knowing your weight is not enough because you may be building muscle without actually losing weight. Muscle ways more than fat so don't be surprised if you're not losing weight. You may still be increasing your muscle size.

You may notice that your weight is the same or that you've actually gained a few pounds during your bodybuilding. However, you may notice that the size of your biceps has increased. By knowing your original weight and measurements, you'll be able to accurately monitor your progress or know if you're actually making progress or need to modify your schedule or routine.

Steps for Successful Workouts

The first thing in any bodybuilding routine is knowing what your goals are and how you wish to achieve them. Based on what you decide, you will determine how many days you wish to train and how many hours per day.

Your basic goal should be to build your biceps and chest muscles. These are the first areas where you'll want to see a difference. You need to put them through a certain amount of stress so they'll grow, making sure to not overdo it. By putting them through a certain stress level, each workout will become easier.

Make sure you give your body plenty of rest between sessions. Many beginners tend to overdo it as soon as they begin to see some progress or if they don't see enough progress. By working the body too hard, they're actually slowing down their progress. Lastly, if you expect to continue to build muscle mass, you need to ensure that your body gets an adequate amount of healthy calories.

In body building, it seems that everyone wants their results the day before yesterday and many are not willing to do what is needed to develop their muscles. Quickly is a relative term. To some it is a week, a month, maybe two months. There are a number of supplements on the market that claim they build muscle fast if you take them and work out. The key is the work out- without that little bit of action no matter what you take legal or illegal the results will be the same- nothing. So research the supplements carefully so you know what you are going to take, if you can try to talk to someone who is using the brand you want to try and see what they think of it. To me, nothing more than a good vitamin supplement and maybe a mineral supplement if there isn't much in the vitamins.

A proper diet full of protein, vegetables, fruits and whole grain carbs is the best thing you can possibly do for yourself. As far as building muscle fast, a lot depends on your own make up too and age the younger you are the easier it will be do build muscle fast. As you are doing this know that you need to fuel these new muscles with lots of healthy foods and plenty of water as well. The body can't build muscle fast is it isn't in top form to begin with. In a month you should see and feel a difference in your body especially if you are eating right along with your build muscle fast weight program. At this point you should add some aerobics for your heart's conditioning too.

Now that you are on track nutritionally, you can begin your weight training. Identify the area that you want to build up the most and work your routine around that area but don't forget the rest of your body, it would benefit as well from toned muscles even if you aren't interested in building the muscles up. You want to work on the arm/back/chest to start out with. Free weights are good because they allow movements that a machine doesn't and can work different groups at once instead of one set at a time with a machine.

Butterflies, one arm lifts, bicep curls these will all be of assistance in your goals with your arms and shoulders. Start with light weight and reps until you are into it then increase the weight and lessen the reps .you can also decrease the time in between then as well for a quicker workout. But keep in mind you can injure yourself easily and be set back to where you started from. Pushups, crunches, squats with weight in your hands they all will help build muscle fast for you.

The best way to tell if you are getting to your goal of building muscle fast is measurements. Hopefully you took them before you started your new routine so you have something to compare it with now. You should see a difference in the numbers on the tape measure. If your waist has actually gone down, this is good. It means the fat around your middle is gone. That is the one place you don't want to see a gain. The scale may tell you that you weight more than you did; this is very possible because muscle weighs more than fat. You will look and feel better with your new healthy body; your mind will function better and be clearer. You will be able to be proud of your accomplishments!

The Origins of Body Building

In the West, it is believed that bodybuilding first came to prominence between 1880 and 1930, when it was promoted by the man who is now often dubbed 'The Father of Modern Bodybuilding', Eugen Sandow.

Indeed, it was Sandow who organized what is generally accepted to be the first ever bodybuilding competition, which he (with commendable understatement) called 'The Great Competition'. This took place at the Royal Albert Hall in London on September 14, 1901, with one of the judges being Sir Arthur Conan Doyle, the writer of the world-famous Sherlock Holmes novels.

Although Sandow did not win the competition, the man who did was presented with a bronze statue of Sandow as his first prize, which is interestingly still given out to the winner of the most prestigious professional bodybuilding competition, Mr. Olympia to this day.

From the 1970s onwards, professional bodybuilding began to be far more organized than previously, with many new organizations such as the International Federation of Bodybuilders (IFBB), and later the National Physique Committee, which according to many is the most successful professional bodybuilding organization in the USA and also acts as the amateur division of the IFBB.

It was also around about the same time that performance enhancing drugs started to become a problem in many sports, and bodybuilding was no exception to this. Back in the 70s, the main drug problem was caused by the use of anabolic steroids by participants in many sports, a problem that was widely discussed and analyzed, because at that time, anabolic steroids were not an illegal substance.

It was probably no coincidence that performance enhancing drugs in bodybuilding started to come to prominence at a time when bodybuilding first began to be recognized as a competitive activity.

Nowadays, anabolic steroids are illegal in most Western countries except when taken under medical supervision. In addition, the list of banned substances is a great deal longer and more detailed than it was back in the 70s, certainly in international sport.

Building a Bigger, Leaner Body

Natural bodybuilding is the very antithesis of building your muscles up using drugs or banned substances, to the extent that 'Natural bodybuilding' means 'bodybuilding without the use of illegal performance enhancing drugs' according to Wikipedia.

One thing to understand about the banned substances that have become a plague on international sport and competition over the past 40 years or so is that most performance enhancers do not really help to enhance performance.

They allow anyone who is training to train harder for a longer period and to recover more quickly. Consequently, by using performance enhancing drugs, it is possible to build up muscle, stamina and fitness far more quickly than if the individual concerned was not abusing these substances.

To anyone who is interested in or is a proponent of natural bodybuilding, the use of artificial substances to help any individual taking part in competition to perform to a higher level than they might otherwise be able to achieve is an anathema.

For this reason, over the past few years, many new natural bodybuilding organizations have been established with the sole purpose of promoting the idea of adding the muscle mass that is necessary for competitive bodybuilding in a totally natural way.

Rather than have an official website of their own, many of these diverse natural bodybuilding organizations have joined together under the one International Natural Bodybuilders Association (but a word of warning – turn your speakers off if you don't want to be deafened by the 'music' that starts playing at deafening volume as soon as you arrive on the homepage!).

On the site, there is a comprehensive list of all substances that are banned in all forms of competition by the World Anti-Doping Agency. Click the link to see the list of substances that are banned as of the 1st of January 2009 in all forms of recognized competition in all sports and activities.

At a competitive or professional level it is therefore clear that banned substances of any form are no longer acceptable in bodybuilding, any more than they are in any kind of recognized sporting activities.

However, the number of people who are professional bodybuilders in comparison to the number of people who are bodybuilders for their own personal enjoyment and satisfaction is extremely small.

Nevertheless, it is not unknown for even the most seemingly laid-back recreational participant in all forms of sport or physical activity to be utterly determined to succeed, and determination of this nature often leads to a temptation to take short cuts.

This is possibly one of the reasons why over the past two or three decades, bodybuilding has (however erroneously) become almost synonymous with participants indulging in banned substances in a desperate effort to attain another 0.1% performance or appearance improvement.

Organizations that actively promote natural bodybuilding like INBA are doing everything they can to banish this impression, but it is often notoriously difficult to change perceptions, and it is slow even if you are successful in doing so.

The bottom line is, while substances that appear on the WADA banned list are there because they enable participants to improve their performance, you should not underestimate the harm and damage that many of these substances can do, particularly if you decide to use them for a period of time.

For example, going back to the favorite performance enhancing drugs of the 1970s, anabolic steroids have a long list of adverse side-effects attached to them. They increase the risk of cardiovascular disease, coronary artery disease, high (bad) cholesterol levels, and high blood pressure and can cause irreparable liver damage.

This is all in addition to other physical problems such as the ability of anabolic steroids to bring on premature baldness in men and to make even women bald (as well as encouraging beard growth in women).

Then there are suspected psychological side-effects such as depression (sometimes leading to suicide), heightened aggression, and a raised risk of developing an addictive personality.

Even some of the natural hormones that are on the WADA banned substances list can have the side-effects, so while it might be assumed that consuming natural hormones will be safe, this is a very general and possibly misguided assumption to make.

For example, Corticotrophins are on the banned WADA list, just one natural hormone selected at random. According to Wikipedia, these are hormones these are produced by the anterior pituitary gland, often in response to stress.

However, they have also been shown to cause mild side-effects such as loss of appetite, worsened acne and diarrhea, as well as far more serious potential side-effects such as severe allergic reactions, muscle pain and weakness, swollen mouth, lips and tongue, and even seizures.

In short, while they may be natural, there are certain levels of human hormones that are 'right' for your body, and 'dosing up' with more significant amounts of a hormone could be potentially dangerous, no matter how natural it might be.

While there is no doubt that the main focus of the WADA list is on prohibiting drugs or substances that enhance performance, it is an inescapable fact that many of these substances can also cause a great deal of harm.

For this reason, it cannot be over emphasized how important it is that no matter how desperate you are to become successful bodybuilder, you do not succumb to the temptation to take performance enhancing substances under any circumstances.

Doing so might at best to be unpleasant but there is also a very significant risk that, especially over the long term, ingesting such substances could be very dangerous indeed.

Chapter 2- The Human Anatomy and How it Reacts to Body Building Efforts

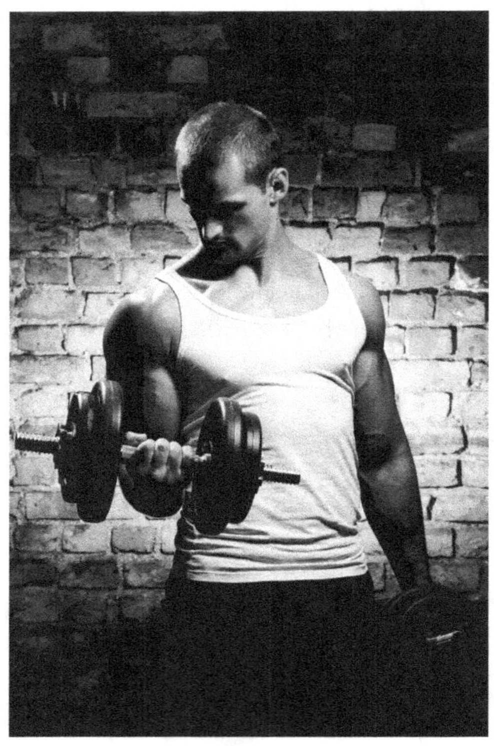

The basic concept of bodybuilding is that bodybuilders (whether professional or amateur) increase their muscle mass while reducing fat levels with the basic objective of looking strong, athletic and generally well-muscled.

In order to achieve their objectives, it is therefore necessary for a bodybuilder to work on developing their musculature. In short, all bodybuilders bulk up their muscle mass until they either start winning the competitions that they enter or until they 'look the way they have always wanted to look'.

However, there is one cloud on this theoretical horizon, which is the fact that no bodybuilder starts with an empty canvas on which they can paint. On the contrary, every bodybuilder starts with the body they have already got, and there is some evidence that the body type and shape that you start with will to an extent dictate how successful you are as a bodybuilder in the future.

To some degree, your success as a bodybuilder is partially genetic; because like any artist or artisan, you can only work with the raw materials you have been given.

There are various genetic factors at work which will to a degree dictate how good a bodybuilder you might become. Let's start to consider some of these factors.

The 3 Body Types

Back in the 1940's, an American numismatist and psychologist Dr. William H. Sheldon propounded the theory that there are essentially three different types of body shape that could cover all men.

As a result of his studies, Sheldon classified all human physiques into one of three categories, which he deemed to be mesomorphs, endomorphs and ectomorphs.

Of the three classifications, the 'kindest' by far, the one that everyone would probably like to be is the mesomorph, which is representative of an individual who has a classic, naturally athletic build. Such an individual would generally be characterized by broad shoulders, a strong back and a large chest. They would be muscular and lean, with above average natural strength.

In other words, a person who could be characterized as a mesomorph is an ideal candidate to be a successful bodybuilder.

An endomorph is a person who is naturally heavy, often someone who has a natural tendency to be fat. An endomorph will often be characterized by a soft, more rounded body shape, a round face and wider hips. It is also quite common for people who are endomorphs to have a naturally heavy bone structure, so it is easy for them to gain weight while difficult to maintain physical fitness.

The ectomorph character is someone who is naturally skinny, with long, thin arms, a slight bone structure, narrow chest and a limited amount of natural body fat.

From the description of the three different types of human physiques that Sheldon recognized, it is going to be easiest for someone who is a mesomorph to become a successful bodybuilder.

However, one thing that has become increasingly clear since Sheldon's original classifications were established is that not everyone fits neatly into one body category or the other. Indeed, some extremely well-known and highly successful amateur and professional competition bodybuilders have exhibited characteristics of more than one classification.

For example, the very first Mr. Olympia Larry Scott was not a particularly metamorphic individual, being noticeably skinny (ectomorph) before he started training to be a bodybuilder. However, by the time he won Mr. Olympia, there is no way that you could suggest that he was skinny, so his body had the ability to 'bulk up'. Larry Scott was an ecto-mesomorph from the beginning, someone who did not fit nicely into one of the Sheldon classifications.

At the other end of the scale, other well-known professional bodybuilders like Danny Padilla were fairly heavily built to start with, and had no problems whatsoever putting on the bulk that they needed to be successful bodybuilders. However, he is believed to have had problems getting lean enough to win competitions, so is forced to follow an extremely rigid diet in order to achieve what he eventually went on to achieve in professional bodybuilding.

In this situation, you could say these individuals were endo-mesomorphs rather than being classic mesomorphs of the type who generally make the best or most natural bodybuilders.

To a certain extent therefore, the type of body you have will have some influence on your body building success. However, even if you are not the perfect mesomorph of the Sheldon classification, it does not follow that bodybuilding is not for you. Whether you could achieve professional status is another question, but I am assuming that you don't want to anyway. At a recreational or personal enjoyment level, bodybuilding is something that almost anyone can do.

There is also another consideration to take into account, which is that other people's perception of us as individuals often affects our attitude to our own body.

For example, if coming to the end of your teens, getting ready to leave home for the first-time, you are the kind of person who has always carried a little weight because Mom's home cooking was just so good, you will probably consider yourself to be just an average guy or girl.

If however everyone starts telling you that you are endomorphic, it is likely that you are eventually going to start pay more attention to other people's opinion of your body type than you do to your own opinions. It then becomes a self-fulfilling prophecy, because if you enjoy your food and you know that you are a naturally fat person (because you've been told this so often), why would you make an effort to change things?

While there is probably nothing intrinsically physiological that prevents you from becoming a successful bodybuilder, psychologically you have already accepted that bodybuilding (and probably every other kind of sport as well) is not for you.

So, while your natural body shape or physique will have some bearing on how successful you are likely to be as a bodybuilder, it is not the be-all-and-end-all. As indicated previously, many highly successful professional bodybuilders were not 'the right shape' by nature, but by dint of hard work and dedication, they became amongst the best in the business.

Perhaps it is fairer to suggest that while their body shape might not have been ideal for becoming bodybuilders, they had metamorphic characteristics somewhere in their makeup that enabled them to become successful in their chosen field. Whether these characteristics were strictly physical or partially physical and partially psychological, it is impossible to say, but if they had these characteristics, there is no reason whatsoever why you may not have them as well.

What about the "Hardgainers"?

The popular perception of a hardgainer is of an individual who can work out regularly with weights for weeks on end and hardly see any improvement in muscle mass other than a slight increase in muscle tone quality.

The classic hardgainer is also most commonly the classic ectomorph, the kind of person that can eat almost anything they want and never put on an ounce of extra weight until they reach the later years of their life when the hormones that control their bodily shape and development are less in control than they were in earlier years.

As previously suggested, being naturally ectomorph does not necessarily mean that you cannot achieve success as a bodybuilder. However, it does mean that you need to approach your bodybuilding development program somewhat differently from the way the classic mesomorph might approach building up their muscle mass.

'How will I Look?'

For anyone who is considering taking up bodybuilding, this is probably one of the first questions that you are likely to ask yourself. While there can never be a definitive answer to this question because to a large extent, the final 'you' will be a result of the amount of work you are prepared to put in, there are many physical characteristics that could have some influence on your final success levels and physical shape.

For example, your body type as already discussed is relevant.

However, to take this analysis one stage further, it is the different components of your body that make up your complete shape, so each of these different parts needs to be considered in isolation to establish how likely it is that you can become a successful bodybuilder.

For instance, your bone structure is extremely important, with the ideal for bodybuilding being wide shoulders and a narrow waist and hips. However, despite the fact that the majority of the most famous bodybuilders do conform to these criteria, not every bodybuilder had naturally wide shoulders and narrow hips.

If you want to become a successful bodybuilder and you do not have the perfect bone structure, it simply means that you have to focus your muscle building activities on developing your body in such a way that it appears that you have ideal bone structure.

Larry Scott was able to create an illusion of the classic V shape torso that is characteristic of successful bodybuilders.

The size and density of your bones is also extremely important for anyone who wants to become a successful bodybuilder, because while strong, heavy bones are a major advantage in full body contact sports like rugby and football, they are not going to be advantageous when your success or failure as a bodybuilder is judged on the way you look.

The opposite is also true. If your skeletal frame is too light and perhaps a little weak, it could limit on the amount of muscle mass you can carry on your frame as well as the amount of weight you can lift in the gym.

Other individual characteristics of bone structure are also important if you want to achieve the perfect bodybuilder pose and look. As an example, a big rib cage as exemplified by Arnold Schwarzenegger is a huge advantage for a bodybuilder, because it naturally creates potential for a bigger chest and greater upper back muscle development.

In a similar manner, the length of your bones makes a difference to the final shape you can achieve, and there is absolutely nothing you can do to change the shape of your bones, so it is a question of working with what you have.

For instance, long legs suggest an ectomorph body area, so they may be more difficult to develop, but long legged bodybuilders naturally look taller.

Then you have the muscles which are the 'building bricks' around which all of your bodybuilding development work will be centered. Many people do not understand that natural muscle shape is a characteristic unique to every individual with the shape itself been dictated by how far the muscle is naturally stretched.

If you have muscles that are attached to the bone at each end quite closely together, you are likely to have fairly compressed muscles which form a noticeable peak when the muscle is tensed. Such big muscles are a big advantage in competitive bodybuilding, which is one of the reasons that Schwarzenegger was so successful (take a look at his biceps to see what I mean).

Others have muscles that are attached much further down the bone, with the attached ends being further apart. In this case, the muscle will demonstrate a considerably smoother, more flowing image, rather than appearing to reach a peak. Again, compare biceps between Schwarzenegger and Larry Scott to see a couple of very good examples of the differences.

What Does All These Entail?

The main thing that you have to take away is that while every individual who decides to become a bodybuilder enters the fray with different 'raw materials', it does not automatically follow that your body shape or bone structure limits what you can do.

However, it is going to be helpful if you can analyze the kind of person you are before starting your bodybuilding training, because knowing what your raw materials are should enable you to approach bodybuilding far more practically. While it is probably not realistic to expect you to understand all of the fine-detail niceties of whether your bone structure is perfect for bodybuilding or not, or whether your muscle attachment points are suitable, you should be able to come up with a general idea of the kind of person you are before embarking on bodybuilding training.

The importance of this is that bodybuilding success ultimately depends on three factors - your general lifestyle, the training program you adopt and proper nutrition.

As we progress through this book, we will look at all of these different aspects of how to become a successful bodybuilder, but only you can know what raw materials you are starting with before you begin doing whatever is necessary to become a bodybuilding success.

CHAPTER 3- THE CAUSES OF BODY BUILDING FAILURE

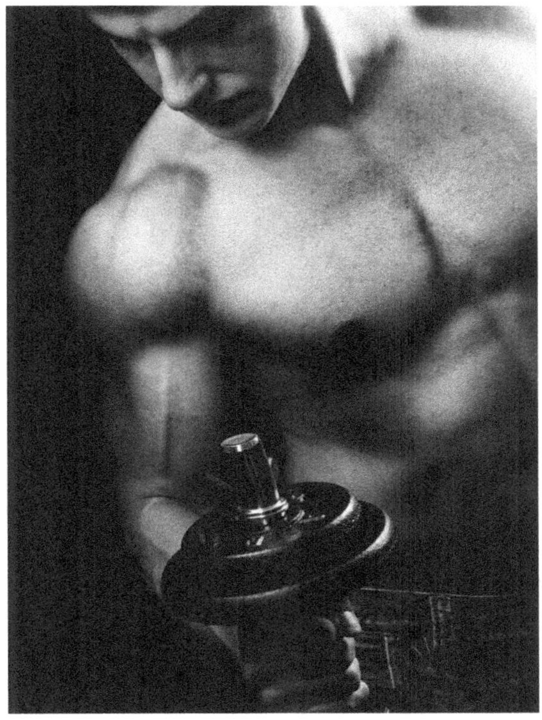

Bodybuilding is a sport that requires hard work, commitment and goals. Sometimes, regardless of how hard a bodybuilder may try, they just seem to fail to meet their goals. They get frustrated and attempt to increase the intensity of the routines, eat more food or perform a number of tasks that actually do more damage than good rather than getting back to the basics. Here are the main reasons why bodybuilders fail to meet their bodybuilding goals.

Not having the right bodybuilding goals is one of the main reasons why bodybuilders fail to succeed. We need goals in every part of our lives. Without goals, we're just going through life aimlessly without a real purpose. In order to be successful at bodybuilding, a bodybuilder needs to know where they want to be when they're finished and what needs to be done to reach that place. They must have a clear picture of what steps need to be taken and in what order to meet their goals. They must never forget these goals.

If you're a bodybuilder that has a professional trainer, you're probably on the right track in knowing what you need to do to meet your bodybuilding goals. Many beginners either go to the gym with no purpose or training plan or start a bodybuilding regimen that's way too strict for a beginner. Both of these scenarios spell disaster and failure in meeting bodybuilding goals. You need to have a specific bodybuilding plan from the first day you begin. Have a purpose.

Many beginning bodybuilders don't realize the importance of a bodybuilding diet. Regardless of what we're doing in life, we need to eat a sensible and well balanced diet. Bodybuilders are no exception. In fact, they need to pay special attention to their diet to ensure they're getting the protein, carbs and other special nutrients they need to help build muscles while keeping up their energy levels.

Now that we're on the subject of diets for bodybuilders, we'll touch on the subject of bodybuilding supplements. You may find that some supplements are very good for your body. However, supplements cannot take the place of good training and a good quality diet. The only time you'll get truly desired results from bodybuilding supplements is when your training and diet are both at adequate levels. If you are considering bodybuilding supplements, it should be only after you've achieved success in your training and diet.

That old saying about no pain no gain is just an old saying and one I feel should be discarded. Usually by the time you've reached the pain level, you've overdone it and have only hurt your progress.

Your body needs the proper amount of rest and recovery between bodybuilding sessions. Without proper rest, your body will not perform as you'd like and your muscles will not grow. Keep in mind that your muscles actually grow when you're sleeping, not when you're working out, as many believe.

The Major No-No's of Body Building

Bodybuilding involves hard work and commitment if you expect to see any real and lasting results. It's important that you use the correct combination of these two things. Here are some simple rules to follow to avoid common mistakes often made by overzealous bodybuilders that can hinder your progress.

- Training too long is not going to give you better results. You shouldn't be putting more than 60 to 75 minutes in at the gym. There is a fine line between an intense workout and overdoing it. Just because a 30 minute workout brings good results doesn't mean doubling it will give twice the results. It will result in sore and tired muscles, which can hinder your progress.

- Not training hard enough can be just as ineffective as overtraining. In order for your muscles to develop, they need stimulation and stimulation comes from pushing them to the point where they can't do any more repetitions.

- Watch your diet. The old myth about eating everything in sight to beef up your body really is just a myth. The key is to eat a well-balanced nutritional diet at all times.

- Get plenty of rest. If you expect your body to perform for you, it needs to be fully rested and ready to go to work. The right amount of sleep for a bodybuilder is at least 8 hours.

- Stick to your basic exercises. It takes time for your body to build muscles and you can't "jump the gun" to bigger exercises without getting the basics out of the way.

- Stay motivated. While it may be easy to become frustrated when you're not getting the results you want in the time you'd hoped, losing motivation will only slow you down more. Know what you want and be willing to work for it.

- Set goals with timelines. It's so easy to allow ourselves to fall into a comfortable routine. Routines are great, but with bodybuilding, you need to have goals so you have something to work towards. Each time you advance to a new exercise, you should have a certain goal in mind.

- Always be competitive. This doesn't mean that you should strive to be the best in the gym, but a good competition will keep you motivated while providing you with goals. Even if it's just yourself you're competing with, you need competition. If there is a competition coming up soon, work towards getting ready for that event.

- Don't skip workouts. You need to be consistent with your exercise routines. Everyone will skip a workout here and there, but repeated missed workouts will hurt you mentally as well as physically.

- Set big goals. Always go for the moon is my motto. Always strive to be better than you are so you don't get set in your ways.

Chapter 4- The Body Building Mindset

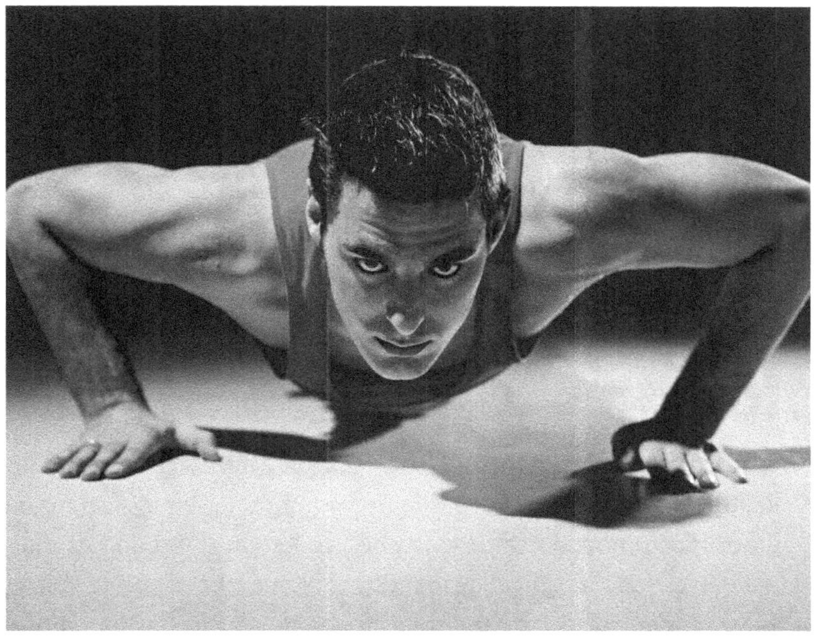

Healthy living is the buzz phrase in today's lifestyle and one of the key areas many people are focused on is getting into shape with admirable and fit bodies. Many people are searching high and low for information on how to get their bodies into good shape. People are keen to lay their hands on any information perceived to be helpful on the subject of healthy living and body shaping. This has opened the gates to various innovations and inventions around health and fitness workout concepts.

The starting point in the efforts to build up your body is to understand that the good looking body is already there, it's just covered under a veneer of fat. Work out programs are designed to help you shape up your body and hence must be tailored to help you wear off the fat and leave your muscles visible right around the key areas of your body. One critical area in the domains of body building is to set on your mind on your goals and make it a point that you are mentally prepared for the task you are about to get into. This is because body building is a discipline which will call for determination, consistency and patience.

The first step in tackling the dynamic of weight loss and body building is to enter into a well laid out and professionally structured program that will enable you to get your body into shape. Getting fit is one of the critically important things if you want to live your life to the fullest. There are many ways of getting fit yet natural weight loss methods have proved to be some of the most effective methods. Being fit generally denotes being in a healthy condition in which one is able to perform ably in physically demanding activities.

There are many indicators of the lack of fitness. One common indicator is running out of breathe in carrying simple physical tasks. The other common indicator is the accumulation of fat and gaining undesirable body weight. These indicators must be taken seriously if the problem of lack of fitness has to be nipped in the bud. Body building calls for an understanding of the fact that the discipline will take some time before some results can be seen. You must then be mentally conditioned for hard work leveraged on the key aspects of determination and patience. Shortcuts such as taking in steroids and other detrimental supplements must be avoided at all costs.

The simple secret to getting fit is consistency. Getting your body involved in regular workouts helps to burn out the calories that amount to the undesirable body weight. Workouts lead to the utilization of these fats and thus lead to a significant reduction of the fat leaving your body trimmed to size, making you appear sexy and healthy. Workouts are not a reserve for the celebrities and models who are keen to maintain lean sexy shapes, they are for everyone especially those who treasure healthy living. Assuming you work out safely there are also no side effects of picking up this healthy habit.

Many people have regarded the objective of staying fit as an objective of models and celebrities who have to carve up good shapes for the cameras or celebrity roles. This is a misconception. Negligence on the aspects of healthy living and physical fitness leads to grave ill health conditions at best and death at worst. Medical researchers have attested to the fact that there is a prevalence of heart related diseases like heart failure, coronary diseases, diabetes and many others which are attributable to unhealthy living. Some of the serious health conditions can be avoided through healthy eating and doing exercise regularly.

Nonetheless there are times when your medical condition is not suitable for health and fitness measures. Medical researchers have shown that when one's health is already compromised in cases where one is already under some form of illness the immune system is already struggling. Doing workouts in this condition is not recommended as it may lead to the deterioration for your immunity condition. However workouts in normal conditions are some of the best natural weight loss methods and also feasible means of boosting your immunity system. To succeed in your body building endeavor you have to set realistic goals. You then have to break these down to smaller achievable objectives. Failure to do this will result in your body building dream towering upon you like a stumbling block. The result is failure and frustration.

Some individuals in keen pursuit of well-shaped bodies and well grown muscles have gotten lured into the temptation of using detrimental health supplements in order to quicken the muscle build-up process. Research has proved that there are detrimental so called health supplements in the market which will compromise your health in the long run. It is wise to seek professional counsel in your health and fitness program. You also have to always remember that the best results in growing your muscles come from the natural methods.

Chapter 5- Tips for the Bodybuilding Beginners

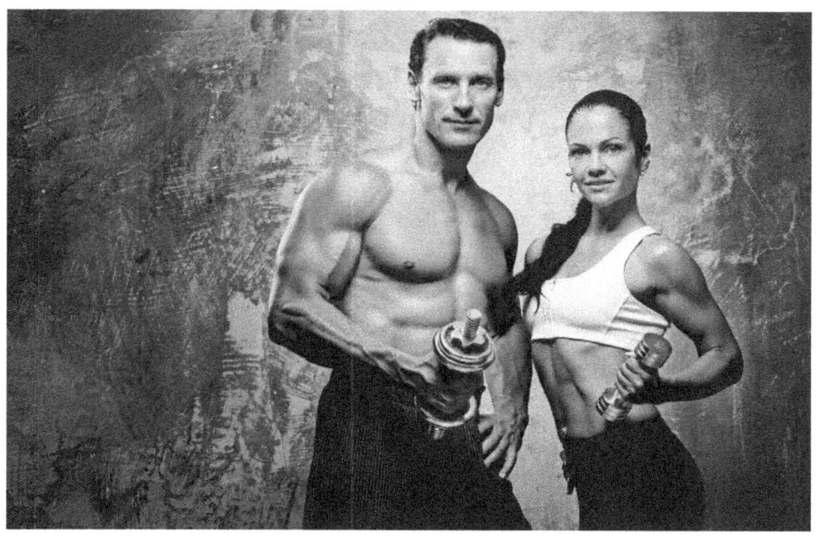

Bodybuilding is a good idea, but not just because it may result in you having the body of your dreams. Bodybuilding is good because along with bodybuilding comes physical exercise and a good healthy diet of well-balanced foots, which are the very things our bodies need to stay healthy.

Many beginners go into bodybuilding headfirst without realizing the importance of the other requirements I mentioned. They believe if they are dedicated to their bodybuilding that's all they need. However, without proper exercise and a good nutritional diet, bodybuilding will not only become difficult, but it may also not lead to the desired results.

Why bother getting into bodybuilding if you're not going to do it right so you'll reach the maximum success? It will only lead to your feeling frustrated and feeling like you failed. Here are a few very important tips for beginners that are interesting in bodybuilding.

Start Slow

Once you've decided you're definitely getting into bodybuilding, you're going to be eager to get right at it so you'll get the fastest results. Here is one thing to always keep in mind. Whether you're overweight or just looking to improve your body, remember that it did not get into the shape it is overnight. Therefore, you're not going to get miraculous results overnight either. You need a lot of patience and you need to start with the basics and be willing to put in the necessary time.

While many beginners get their research for bodybuilding online or from friends, others seek the help of a professional trainer. If this is within your budget, it's a great idea because a trainer can show you the best bodybuilding steps, while allowing you to work at your pace. Working at your own pace and not overdoing it is the most important thing.

Males vs. Females

Many women see a man's body in a bodybuilding magazine and feel they can easily achieve the same goal by doing the same bodybuilding exercises and using the same techniques. What's important to remember is that a woman's body is built differently than a man's to start with. Secondly, factors like pregnancy, menstruation, nursing and even menopause take a toll on a woman's body and special considerations need to be taken. These considerations are not just the required bodybuilding techniques but also the different nutritional requirements.

Nutrition

Don't ever underestimate the importance of a well-balanced diet, whether you're bodybuilding or not. There are many supplements you can take, but if your body is lacking the nutrition it needs, your progress is not going to be what you want. It's also important that your diet meet the requirements of your body, as everyone's needs are different.

Good Bodybuilding Habits Mean Successful Bodybuilding

Whether you're just beginning bodybuilding or have been at it for a while now, you've probably been given many bodybuilding tips. Some may be guaranteed to help your reach your goals quicker, others may be exercise tips and others may just be ways to make your bodybuilding more enjoyable.

Regardless of what type of tips you've received, you're probably not sure which ones to take to heart. The most important thing to remember is that without good bodybuilding habits, you will not be successful at your bodybuilding. There's no big secret for success. It's all back to the basics. By practicing good bodybuilding habits, you'll have more fun and reach your fitness goals much quicker.

- Dress appropriately. You are not at a fashion show so make sure your clothing allows free movement. If you're a male, wear a t-shirt. As proud of your abs as you may be, no one should have to see and smell your armpits!

- Drink plenty of water before, during and after each workout. Water is the healthiest beverage you can put in your body. It will also help with weight loss. Regardless of how many fitness beverages you'll find on the market, nothing is as good as water, even when you're not working out.

- Always warm up before you begin lifting weights. Whether you choose to go on a treadmill for a few minutes, ride a stationary bike or do several good stretches, just make sure you warm up before your sessions begin. Failure to warm up properly can result in some very sore muscles, which can slow down your bodybuilding process. A good warm up may consist of a few cardio exercises followed by weights that are about 40% lighter than what you use in your sessions.

- Make sure you lift properly. There is more to lifting than just bending down and picking something up. The old saying about lifting with your legs rather than your back really is true. Incorrect lifting techniques can result in damaged ligaments and tendons, torn muscles or worse.

- Concentrate on what you're doing. Regardless of how impressive the bodybuilder next to you may be, pay attention to what you're doing. Losing concentration is a sure recipe for injury. If you are interested in his or her techniques or progress, wait until you've finished your session to carry on a conversation.

- Eat a good diet. Few things are as important to your bodybuilding goals as eating a well-balanced nutritional diet. This will help you to be more successful at weight loss as well as muscle building.

CHAPTER 6 – HOW TO SHAPE UP YOUR BODY ASSETS

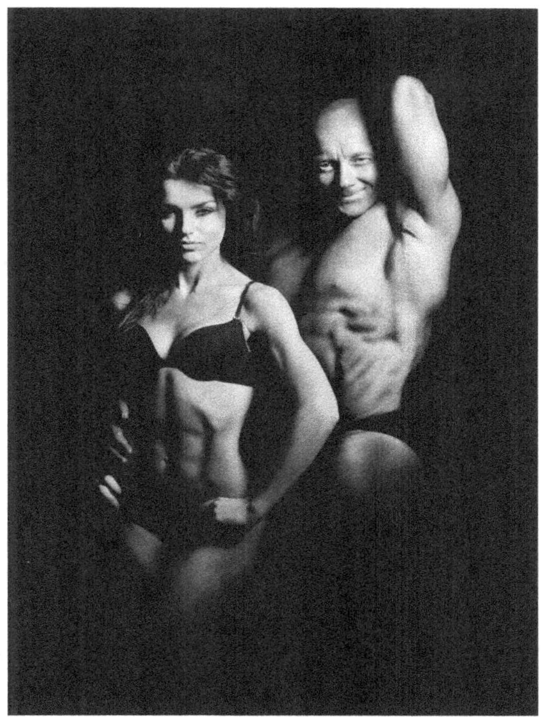

• Toning the Belly

Accumulating unwanted stomach fat is one common phenomenon for teenagers, youths and adults alike. There have been various ways presented in an effort of fighting stomach fat yet not all these ways are effective. Natural weight loss measures are the best option to put up a good fight against belly fat. Belly fat occurs in the deeper areas of the body which is in contrast to subcutaneous fat (fat that accumulates under the skin). Stomach fat is a serious condition since the fat accumulates around critical organs that are in the abdomen. There is a resonating concern between high body fat and the prevalence of fat related diseases such as heart and coronary diseases among other fat related deteriorations such as diabetes.

One of the feasible natural weight loss ways of fighting stomach fat is eating 5 to 6 times a day. You may think to yourself, "but this can actually lead to a development of a pot belly'. The catch is that when people stick to the traditional three meals-a-day pattern there is a tendency to binge. Having 5 to 6 smaller meals a day works well as a natural weight loss method because when you take light meals in well slotted intervals you will be less tempted to guzzle down disproportionate amounts of food. The 5-6 meals a day approach is a practical way of avoiding overeating and enhances as well as boosts metabolic processes.

The other natural fat or weight loss approach which has been proved to pay off is the intake of the kinds of foods that burn fat. Empirical research has proved that foods that have high levels of protein and low components of carbohydrates, sugar as well as saturated fats are effective in fighting stomach fat. In pursuing a diet of such foods like lean meats, vegetables and wholesome grains one must also avoid the kind of refined foods that have fine carbohydrates especially those with white sugar. Foods which also contain white flour must be avoided or at least minimized in these natural weight loss methods.

Fighting belly fat takes a holistic approach which enlists various methods such as drinking recommended fluids and plenty of water, weight lifting and doing some cardio workouts. The main focus in fighting stomach fat is about burning the calories and doing a lot of exercise in a realistic way that compliments a good diet. Diet and nutrition has to precede the actual body building workouts and training.

• How to Get Hot Abs Fast

In the modern health conscious society getting good looking abs is a dream worth working towards for most men and women. It is important to get a good package of information before committing your energies, time and financial resources into any fitness and health program. This is even true for abs developing fitness programs. In this section we will share with you some techniques that you can implement to get admirable abs really fast. The development of abs requires a balanced integration of cardiovascular exercises, as well as healthy eating, and abdominal workouts. The secret to abs is not in the ab workouts but in achieving a low body fat to get them visible.

Healthy eating is a must for anyone seeking to trim their body into good shape. The same is true for anyone seeking to get their abs exposed in that admirable awe. When engaged in weight loss body building endeavors it is wise to stay away from refined and highly processed foods. It is good to settle for organic food or wholesome foods which are still in their natural state or close to it. There are no shortcuts on the path of getting anything worthwhile hence you have to understand that getting that abs faster still entails some discipline and consistency on your part.

The other critical dynamic around eating healthily is to get out of the three heavy meals routine and settle for about 5-6 light meals a day. The more the better as you will be activating your metabolism more frequently. This also ensures that you do not get into excessive hunger which may prompt you to crave. The key thing to remember is that these meals are small. Usually 350-550 calories if you are a man and 250-450 if a woman. When you get into the condition of excessive hunger you are then mostly likely to guzzle and this will result in eating way over needed proportions and this has been one of the major causes of obesity. Eating in-between meals also ensures that your body always has enough energy thus prompting your metabolism to burn out those unwanted calories.

The other critical component of developing abs in your health and fitness program is to ensure that your exercises will heavily involve your abdominal muscles. Whilst you are also so keen to ensure that you are getting rid of that fat make sure your workouts and your diet are adding more tissue onto your body. It is also imperative to get your body into cardiovascular conditioning through well designed exercises and other workouts. These methods are essential in your dream of getting good abs into shape. Remember you can strengthen your abs through abdominal exercises, but the only way to get them to show is by lowering fat. This means abs is built in the kitchen along with the cardio machine.

- **Building Your Upper Body Muscles**

People have associated great body shaping and body building results with going to the gym. The reality is that there are some workouts that you can conduct in the comfort of your home and without any equipment whatsoever to get remarkable results. This is especially true for the objective of building and shaping up the upper body. In this section you will get an outline of some easy-to-follow guidelines on how to get your body into good shape without going to the gym and forking out money to purchase expensive equipment.

1. Push-ups. This is one of the easiest yet effective set of exercises you can do in the comfort of your home. Like any other fitness and body building endeavors these have to be done the right and effective way otherwise your efforts will amount to waste and frustration. If you do these the right way you will be on your way to accumulate the desired pecs, shoulders, triceps that you see in fitness magazines. Make sure you complete the exercise in a full

range of motion to engage all the muscles needed to perform a proper push-up. If regular push-ups are too hard for you, you can always attempt modified pushups (with your knees on the ground and your shins pointing up making a 45 degree angle) until you build up more upper body strength.

2. Pull-up. This one is one of the highly effective exercises of building your back. You will have to find something like a long vertical pole somewhere in your yard that you can sustain yourself up with. Make sure that you drop all the way down on a pull up and pull yourself up above the chin. This full range of motion will target your lats and back muscles like never before.

3. The Triceps-Dip. This one deals with developing your triceps muscles head on. In this exercise you have to use your chair and place your hands behind you as well raise the lower section of your body whilst forcing arms to lift your body weight. Also you have to do this exercise using proper technique and working to stretch your muscles to the furthest possible limit. This way you are sure to be working your way right through to a position where you will develop stronger arms.

- **Getting a V-Shaped Back**

There are countless programs and products for sale in the market promising to offer remarkable makeovers. Truth of the matter is that not many of these flaunted programs and products are easily effective as far as what they claim to achieve is concerned. Before committing your finances and time to any fitness product or program you need to do some wide research and consultation which will help you establish the best health and fitness program and products that suit your custom body condition and needs. A stern and muscular back is one of the strongly coveted merits of health and fitness programs. In this section we will share with you three feasible back shaping exercises which can be done easily from home to earn you that admirable muscular back.

One of the methods involves the use of the Incline Dumbbells. With this method you need to sit backwards and have your chest pressed on an incline bench. This activity can be done with a pair of dumbbells. In doing this you need have yours arms hang vertically towards the floor then you have to inhale as you raise the dumbbells straight up in the direction of your sides. You will have to keep in this position for about a second and then drop the angle of your arms to the starting point. You have to complete a set of eight of these continuously.

The second method entails the use of Barbell Rows. In this method you have to bend and grip the barbell with both hands. Here you have to keep your knees almost straight and just slightly bent. With this method you have to keep your feet shoulder width and avoid moving your knees or leg during this exercise. Your focus must remain on the back. You then have to inhale and lift the barbell to your chest with your head facing the floor in front of you and then place the barbell back to the floor. A set of eight of these repeated 4 times would make it for a day.

The last method is very effective for those who would want to develop a good looking V-shaped torso. These methods entail the use of pull bars. This exercises mainly involve the grasping the bar at various dimensions and angles with arms fully extended. Various stunts as outlined in different training packages will help you get the best results floor of the pull bar back muscles building programs.

CHAPTER 7 – BUILDING THE CORE MUSCLES

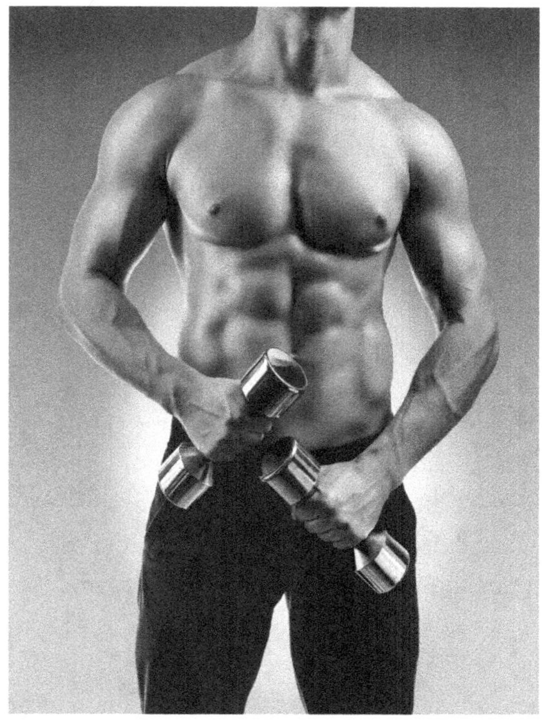

Many fitness programs focus almost invariably on workouts programs aimed at building muscles and trimming the body into good shape. Good as it is this has often led to the neglect of other important dynamics and dimension of maintaining a healthy body and lifestyle. One area that has been neglected and has had less said about is the aspect of strengthening core muscles. The strengthening of core muscles is a critical aspect of any health or fitness endeavor. Your core muscles are in your back and the abdominal. These have to be kept in good and stern shape as well as positioning. Without this your body will slump into shapelessness and it is important that before you get into any serious body building regimen that your core muscles are conditioned. Keeping your core muscles in good condition will give you that stern and bold God-given stature upon which you can then enhance the size and shape of your muscles to get that lean and muscular body.

The building of core muscles is a must-do for all body builders and weight lifters. This is due to the fact that the core muscles play a crucial and irreplaceable role in sustaining the weight of your body when you conduct all forms of workouts. It is the role of the core muscles to keep your body in good balance. Many body builders focus on weight loss and forget about keeping the core muscles strong and stern. The result of the neglect is that the core cannot sustain the weights that the lifter attempts and this increases the chance of injury.

Various forms of works outs are designed for certain muscles groups like the chest, biceps and triceps etc. and many work out structures neglect the strengthening of the core muscles in the back and in the abdominal. Some body builders may develop well shaped muscles and bodies but have problems or sometimes injuries associated with lifting certain objects. This is due to the fact that the body builder has focused on say, building biceps but the rest of the core muscles in the back have not been strengthened to cope with heavy weight lifting. Dancers are good at working at their core muscles that is why they can perform stunning stunts in dance.

CHAPTER 8 – BODY BUILDING EXERCISES

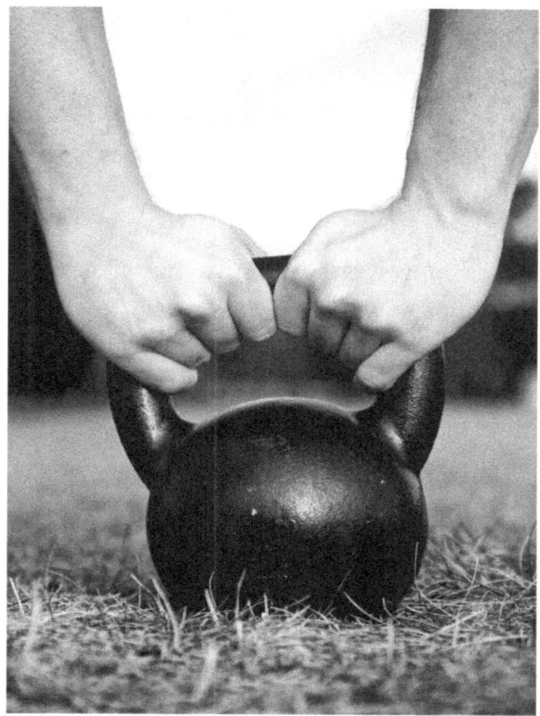

Compound Exercises

The thing is with compound exercises there is a higher risk involved for the lifter. When you are doing compound exercises you have to ensure that your form is correct and you need to have a spotter, especially when you attempt heavier weights. There is a bunch of different type of compound exercises but some of the best to perform are bench press, squats, deadlifts, barbell rows, and military press.

Bench Press – The bench press is the preferred exercise for building powerful pectoral muscles. The triceps and shoulders are also involved to some degrees. Many people manipulate different angles (incline/decline) to target different muscle areas but in my experience the flat bench press is adequate enough. If you are new to bench pressing, it's imperative to get your form down as the bench press is an exercise that is tricky to master. I would recommend choosing a weight that you can push to 10-12 reps as a beginner before moving on to heavier weight / less rep routines. To start on the bench press make sure your head is at the top of the bench. When taking the bar off the rack make sure that it is directly above your chest.

The bench press movement is simple but it is hard to control especially under heavy weight. You want to slowly bring the bar down to the middle of your chest (all the way down to your chest, you may see some people in your gym going ½ way but I assure you they are wasting their time as this is not a full press) and push up in a straight line. The shortest distance between two points is in a straight line, so do not tilt or move the bar, have it go straight down to your chest and push straight up without locking out. It may help to envision your feet pushing into the floor to help gain leverage. You do not want your back arching on the bench press and your shoulder blades should for the most part be on the bench at all times.

Good growth follows good form so if you have to sacrifice weight in order to do the proper movement, and then lose the ego. A few weeks of proper benching will ensure growth for even the hardest of gainers.

Squats – A lot of people avoid squats because it's an exercise that will leave your legs sore for days. Besides being one of the most beneficial compound movements, squats will work your core like no other exercise so it's extremely important that you master them. A lot of time when people do squats, they do them incorrectly. When squatting, you have to go what is known as "parallel". This means that your butt goes down far enough that the angle of your calves and hamstrings go past 90 degrees. When squatting, keep your back straight and your stomach tucked. When you squat down it is important to breathe in, and slowly let the air out as you go back up. Do not lock out your knees at the end of your squat motion, try to keep the movement as fluid as possible (which means you should try not to "rest" at the bottom of the movement as well). Squats are a tough exercise, but for good reason.

As a beginner, it will be hard to go all the way down parallel, but keep pushing yourself and the flexibility will soon come. Squats not only work your quads, hamstrings, glutes and more but they also condition your lower back and abdominals. If you want to improve your core strength then squats is the exercise that simply needs to be put in your arsenal.

Deadlifts – One of my personal favorite exercises are the deadlifts. Even though dead lifts work out the hamstrings to a major degree, I like to do them on a back day. I save squats for legs and space out my dead lift day far enough so my legs are properly recovered. Many people perform the dead lifts in a similar fashion to a "reverse-squat". This is not the correct way to deadlift. To begin the movement, the barbell should be rubbing against your shins. Your legs should be spaced a little more than shoulder width apart and you need to look straight ahead.

As you squat down to lift up the bar make sure your knees are not going too far past the barbell. Use your hips to pull the weight back up as well as lifting your back straight at the end of the movement. Like all the other exercises, the movement needs to be fluid; there should not be a pause, or two distinct separate movements. An overhand grip will also strengthen your forearms, but if you find that your grip is stopping you from lifting heavier weights you can always invest in a pair of weight lifting straps or use a one hand overhand, one hand underhand grip. Deadlifts will help you get the v-shaped back you always wanted and will strengthen a majority of your muscles in your body.

Barbell Rows – Barbell Rows are a great way to target your lats, and your deltoids depending on how you position yourself. To begin the exercise have your knees slightly bent, look straight ahead and with your back straight and chest high up pull your elbows in without moving. If you find yourself moving your back or chest, you will not be isolating the proper muscles for the movement and you will not effectively strain the muscle for adequate growth. Keep your body locked in besides your arms when you bring your elbows back. Have a trainer watch over your form so you are training the appropriate muscles. When you are pulling the bar back it should reach a few inches above your navel but not as high to reach your chest.

Military Press – Military Presses are one of the best exercises you can do for your shoulder muscles. If you prefer, you can use dumb-bells as well. The military press starts off with you being on an incline flat bench. Your back should be straight and your legs should be planted on the ground. What you want to do is grab the barbell about 1.5x shoulder width and make sure that your grab the barbell tight, you want it to be resting in your hand but not pulling back on your wrist. Lift the barbell a few inches above your head then slowly bring it back down to about eye/nose position. Do this for a few reps while maintaining a good posture and well controlled movements. Military presses will pound your shoulders like no other exercises so it's important to do them well.

There are other compound movements that you can complete as a bodybuilder such as clean and jerks. In my opinion, these compound movements are usually more risky and if you are not a professional you should not even think about attempting them. The 5 compound movements listed above will work every major muscle group in your body, and they are safe to practice as long as you maintain strict form and have a spotter watching over you.

Another thing on form is that it takes years to perfect, so as a beginner you want to start off with low weights just until you can build the mind to muscle connection that these exercises employ. It may be hard to set aside your ego for proper form, but trust me, in a few months down the line your body will thank you. I see guys in my gym all the time pushing around weights like they own the place, but their forms are horrendous, and I doubt they could even do ½ of what they shoot for with proper technique. Your ego is your biggest enemy in your bodybuilding endeavors so leave it outside and make sure to master the movements properly before you attempt to lift heavier weights.

Aerobic Exercises

Bodybuilding involves more than just heavy and rigorous training on exercise machines, although this is a large part of what bodybuilding is all about. The warm up you give your body before your workout is every bit as important as the bodybuilding exercises.

Aerobic exercises are often used as a form of warming up for bodybuilding as well as an excellent form of exercise on their own. Many people that are unfamiliar with exercise and training don't always know what aerobic exercise is all about and how important it is to our overall good health.

What is Aerobic Exercise?

Aerobic exercise is very important for our body because it will keep our bodies trim and fit. However, it's also an excellent form of exercise for your cardiovascular system. Just, what is aerobic exercise? Any time you're doing any exercise that has you breathing harder than normal and makes your heart rate increase is aerobic exercise. You may have many aerobic exercise groups in your area. However, you don't have to be part of an exercise group to reap the many benefits of aerobic exercise.

Benefits of Aerobic Exercise

In addition to the benefits aerobic exercise provides for our heart, it is also an excellent option for burning fat. Our bodies consist of two energy sources. One source is sugar and the other is fat. Sugar, which is our easiest form of energy our body can use, is stored in our muscle and liver. Although fat can be used for energy, it requires more work for us to use it. The reason for this is that fat is only broken down if there is available oxygen.

We need oxygen to allow our bodies to burn fat for energy, but it is not needed to burn sugar. When we first begin exercising, oxygen is not available. It isn't until we've been exercising for at least 30 minutes that fat can be used by our muscles as a source of fuel.

Aerobic exercise enhances our blood flow, which improves oxygen level so our body can build more muscle. This is the most important reason why aerobic exercise should be a part of our lives, whether exercising for fun or as part of bodybuilding. It's not only excellent for our hearts but has many other health benefits. Aerobic exercise will help to speed up your metabolism, which will help you to lose weight. It's also great for lowering your blood pressure, which has many health benefits.

When you first begin aerobic exercise, you may want to start with just 5 to 10 minutes and work your way up to sessions of at least 20 minutes. Some excellent choices of aerobic exercise include jogging or biking.

Weight Training

One of the great things about using the internet for 'learning' is that there are some subjects where the net happens to be the perfect medium to pick up all of the information you could ever need.

Weight training for bodybuilding is one terrific example of this, because by the very nature of body building, it is a 'sport' that is focused on looking good.

Consequently, there are hundreds of bodybuilding enthusiasts on the net who are more than happy to show off exactly how they got to where they are today, which presents you with an 'open window' through which you can learn from other people who have already 'been there and done that'.

Run any kind of net search for weight training for bodybuilding information, and there is a ton of stuff available for free.

Even more importantly, because many of the weight training educational materials are available on video, it is not just a question of reading about what people do, you can watch them as they train. Most people find that watching is far more educational than reading about something, so this is a major bodybuilding advantage that was not available to our forebears.

The basic idea of weight training for bodybuilding is that you need to focus on developing the muscle groups that need most development for you to acquire the shape that you want to acquire.

Going back to an earlier example to highlight this point, you may remember that Larry Scott spent a great deal of time working on developing his deltoid and pectoral muscles to gain the shape that he wanted, because these were the muscles that he needed to develop to create a 'fake' V-shape that is (or was) the classic bodybuilding shape.

You need to do the same thing by designing a weight training program that focuses on the muscles you most want to develop.

While for many bodybuilders this will mean focusing on the muscles of the upper torso and waist area, it does not follow that this will always be the case. For example, there have been competition bodybuilders who have had to spend a great deal of time on developing muscles in their legs, because they were people who had great muscle development in the upper half of the body, but very skinny legs!

There is also the question of why you are body building in the first place. If you are developing a physique for your own satisfaction and fitness, then your objectives may well differ from those of a competition bodybuilder who has to attain a body shape that satisfies objective judges, rather than themselves.

In short, your weight training program should be designed to achieve what you want to achieve, but even a quick online survey of the instructional materials available should enable you to find weight training exercises that will satisfy your own requirements extremely effectively.

Chapter 9 – The Body Builder's Diet

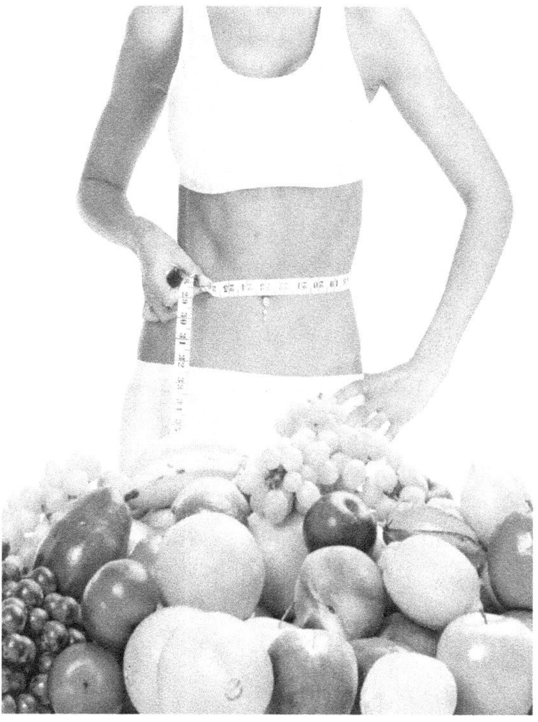

At the heart of natural bodybuilding, the two main things that really count are the amount of effort that you put into your training, and nutrition.

Now, the word 'diet' is often used as a dirty word, especially by people who are trained to lose weight and associate the word with starvation and being deprived of all the things that they most enjoy eating. While adopting a particular diet for bodybuilding purposes is not about starving or even denying yourself your favorite foodstuffs, there is a similar amount of discipline required as would be necessary if you were trying to lose weight.

Building a Bigger, Leaner Body

Let us start by looking at the basics of nutrition for anyone who wants to start bodybuilding, or is interested in doing so more effectively.

The Correct Body Building Nutrition

More is better: One of the first things that you have to do if you are going to adopt a diet regime that is designed to increase muscle mass is to move away from the traditional three meals a day scenario. Instead, you need to eat perhaps five smaller meals a day, with considerably less time in between eating times.

The reason that you do this is that under normal circumstances, your body will assume that there is no more food coming if you don't feed it for more than three or four hours.

Consequently, in this catabolic state, your body will immediately start to feed on lean muscle (leaving your body fat untouched) on the basis that this body fat is high in calories and therefore represents an excellent source of long-term energy if there is no more food coming for a longer period.

This is completely contrary to what you want as a bodybuilder, so you must eat several smaller meals a day, with no more than 2½ or 3 hours between each one.

Balance is the key: When people decide that they want to become bodybuilders, they do not each do so for the same reasons. For example, some people may need to pay more attention to losing fat before starting to build real muscle mass, while others who have already got themselves to a position where their body fat levels are very low will be the opposite, wanting to focus on muscle building right from the very beginning.

Hence, there is an element of your diet having to be focused on whatever it is you specifically want to achieve at this time.

As a general rule, every meal that you take should be balanced between the three micronutrients that every bodybuilder needs, which are proteins, carbohydrates and good fats, with each being taken in the right proportions.

What you should not do is have meals where everything or almost everything you eat falls into the same micronutrient category.

For example, a meal that is made up of little other than carbohydrates (e.g. a bowl of pasta and plain bread with a sliver of spread) is not likely to be a great help to your body building diet, because every meal should attain the balance that you need to achieve your objectives.

As a broad guideline, most body building experts recommend a diet that is 40% carbohydrate, 40% protein and 20% good fats. But the most important thing is, try to make sure that whatever balance you are aiming for, every meal is approximately the same.

Why the glycemic index is important: The glycemic index (GI) is a measure of how quickly your blood sugar levels rise after ingesting a carbohydrate, which always happens because as soon as you take in carbohydrates, it gets turned into glucose. In turn, glucose makes ATP, which is a natural substance that 'drives' everything your body does.

According to the glycemic index, every foodstuff or beverage you ingest is assigned a value, which indicates how quickly sugar is released into your blood after taking that food or drink.

Some substances would act very quickly to increase blood sugar level, if for example you drank a pure sugar drink. Hence, this drink would have a high glycemic index near the upper limit of 100, whereas whole wheat spaghetti has a GI figure of somewhere between 35 and 40.

Given that carbohydrates generate energy for your body, you might assume that the higher the GI figure is for particular foodstuff, the better it will be for anyone who is trying to power their bodybuilding efforts, but you would be wrong. This is because when any food or drink you take in is very high in sugar, it prompts a sudden surge of pancreatic activity to produce insulin.

Unfortunately, while your body is still heavily laden with insulin, it is not capable of losing fat, because the natural hormonal imbalance that has been generated triggers fat storage.

Foods and drinks that have lower GI figures are far better for anyone who is an active bodybuilder, because the release of sugar is naturally slower and therefore the surge of insulin is far more controlled as well.

This means that there are fewer 'highs' and 'lows' and that your appetite is likely to be far more controlled which minimizes the risk of suffering 'snack attacks'.

Lower glycemic index foodstuffs are extremely effective for controlling the amount of fat that you put on, while they also help bulk up your muscles and burn existing fat at the same time.

In a perfect scenario, all you would need to know about the carbohydrate you're eating would be the glycemic index, but nothing is perfect. There are a couple of reasons you cannot use GI as the only guide of how good particular carbohydrates are in your body building diet.

Firstly, if you take on board carbohydrates as well as proteins and fats in the same meal (as we have already established that you should) then both the proteins and fats will slow down the energy absorption from the carbohydrate.

Secondly, there are different types of carbohydrate and they are handled in different ways by the body.

On the one hand you have complex carbohydrates such as starchy foodstuffs like oatmeal, sweet potatoes and lentils, while on the other there are fibrous carbohydrates such as asparagus, broccoli, cauliflower and tomatoes. If you eat a combination of starchy and fibrous carbohydrates together, then the latter slows down the absorption of the former, thereby lowering their GI rating, which is better for building muscle and reducing fatty deposits.

Eat these compact carbohydrates in small portions at every meal, but make sure that there is a least one portion with every meal.

Whereas complex carbohydrates release energy into the body slowly, simple carbohydrates will do so much more quickly, so foodstuffs like apples, pears, oranges, peaches and strawberries will give you a far quicker energy boost.

The glycemic index is a measure of the power of food to increase blood glucose levels after consumption. The more power you take in, the more power needs to be burned off if you are going to attain the perfect shape and physique for bodybuilding purposes, whether this is for competition or purely for your own satisfaction.

Building a Bigger, Leaner Body

A bodybuilding diet plan for the early stages: As suggested previously, one of the first things you must do if you are attempting to adopt a diet plan that is to build muscle mass without adding too much additional fat to your frame is to move from the traditional 'three square meals a day' concept to a situation where you eat more regularly, but far less food is taken at every meal.

It is essential to understand that there is a huge industry out there which is actively and often very aggressively pushing supplements of one form or another as the 'cure all' answer that is going to make you into a champion bodybuilder overnight.

The first thing to say about some of these supplements is that they are not all necessarily bad. For example, some meal replacement supplements such as Prolab Lean Mass Complex offer an excellent way of replacing at least one meal every day with a simple to prepare but protein packed instant meal that also features only low glycemic carbohydrates.

However, there are also a lot of supplements of more dubious provenance on the market, and in most cases, it really is not necessary to spend a great deal of money on supplements of this nature.

Successful bodybuilding is a science like anything else, a combination of a successful training program and a diet that is specifically focused on building muscle mass while keeping extraneous fat to a minimum.

A diet that is ideal for a bodybuilder is very little different from the kind of diet that you would expect any high performance athlete to adopt. Irrespective of whether your bodybuilding efforts are aimed at competition or only at personal satisfaction, the same rules still apply. Eat an athletic diet, keep training, and you will inevitably acquire the shape and physique you are looking for.

It is also important to understand that, while there are many extremely popular 'diet plans' such as the South Beach diet, the Atkins diet and more recently, the Jenny Craig diet, a diet for activity (or perhaps more accurately, extreme activity in the case of bodybuilding) is significantly different because while all of these diets focus on reducing fat, none of them are particularly focused on building muscle mass.

Your diet for bodybuilding is likely to be far less strict about what you can and cannot eat, but much broader and all-encompassing than any of these weight-loss-only diet plans. Remember that as a bodybuilder, someone who works out on a regular basis as a part of a preplanned program of muscle building, you cannot afford to be tired or lethargic, whereas it is an unfortunate fact that diet plans which focus only on weight loss can often leave you feeling this way.

Hence, the basis of your body building diet should be focused on the following characteristics and ideas:

• Eat plenty of green vegetables and fresh fruit, while including other essential foods such as whole grains, nuts, pulses, beans and seeds. The odd portion of occasional lean meat is acceptable, while fish, eggs and low-fat dairy products should also be included in your daily eating regime.

• Mono-saturated and polyunsaturated oil products should be included, while saturated fats such as those found in spreads, margarine and in most deep-fried foods should be avoided.

- You should limit your intake of alcohol, cholesterol, salt and any foods or drinks that contain non-natural or added sugar. For instance, while fruit juices which contain natural sugars are acceptable, soda and other similar soft drinks that are fortified with additional sugar should be avoided.

- Do not be tempted by apparently low-sugar soft drinks where the sugar has been replaced with artificial sweeteners. Besides the fact that many artificial sweeteners are of questionable safety, they are generally manufactured from various forms of chemical based solutions, some of which may appear on various banned substance lists.

- Drink plenty of water. For the average person who is 'dieting' (i.e. trying to lose weight), the normal recommendation is for a minimum of eight glasses of water a day, but given that a significant part of your body building efforts is going to be focused on training and exercise, you should 'up' this minimum daily requirement as necessary. Remember that it is almost physically impossible to drink too much water (it is just about possible to damage yourself by trying to drink many, many liters of water at the same sitting, but why would you do this?), so drinking as much water as you want makes a great deal of sense.

Once again, the perfect diet for you as in individual bodybuilder will depend upon your primary objective as a bodybuilder, and your current physical condition as well.

For example, for every foodstuff or beverage you take in, there is a 'Recommended Daily Intake' that is agreed between various government bodies, and the scientific and medical communities.

The actual numbers tend to vary slightly from country to country, but the general picture that comes out of countries like the USA,

Canada, the UK and Australia are all very similar in terms of how much of each different type of foodstuff you need for a continual healthy lifestyle.

Working with these averages will give you an idea of the kind of diet you need to in order to achieve the objectives which you have set yourself.

For example, if you are in the early stages of bodybuilding, where losing fat is the primary objective, then your diet should be aimed at creating an energy deficit.

Fat is nothing more than stored energy that you have consumed at some time in the past that was not burned off, so in order to lose that fat, you need to reverse the process that put it there in the first place. You need to consume 15% to 20% less energy than you need.

However, there is a fairly tricky balancing act to be maintained here, because if you are trying to lose fat while also building muscle mass, you are actually asking your body to do two things which are completely opposite to one another as far as your metabolism is concerned. The act of breaking down the fat is called catabolism, which is one process, while the building up muscle is called anabolism, which is almost diametrically opposite.

If left to its own devices in the event of an energy deficit induced by diet, your body will start to break down fat to provide the missing energy, but it will also try to burn muscle.

This is one reason why weight training is such an essential part of body building activity. By continuing to train while reducing your energy intake, you effectively prevent your body focusing on muscle as a source of energy. Consequently, your body is forced to look elsewhere for its energy source - meaning that after the 'fast burn' glycogen that is the first source of energy your body always turns to, it then turns to burning fat because weight training protects your muscles.

Indeed, it is now believed that even at rest, the more muscle you have, the more your body will focus on burning fat as an energy source.

If you are still in the initial bodybuilding stage where getting rid of fat is your primary consideration, it is still critical to take up weight training as soon as possible. In doing so, you ensure that your body 'burns' the parts that you want it to burn, rather than it doing what comes naturally, looking for energy wherever it might be found.

A diet plan for the later stages: Once you have shifted a significant amount of the fat that you want to get rid of, you are ready to move on to the next stage of your body building diet plan, but before you do, here is something to understand.

In the initial stages, you reduce the amount of energy you are consuming to below the minimum of what you really need as a way of prompting your body to use stored fat to make up the energy deficits.

You have managed to get rid of most of this fat, but you should not try to get rid of all body fat before moving on to the next phase. This is because during this next phase, you are going to reverse the previous eating program by eating more than you need. The primary objective of this is to build additional muscle mass, but it is also an inevitable side effect that you will also generate some additional body fat.

In this next 'bulking up' phase, you should aim to consume around 15% to 20% more energy than an average person of your size and weight needs to get through the average day.

You can either guess on this, or you can use a size and weight calculator to get a more accurate picture of what you need to eat every day to satisfy your muscle building requirements.

In terms of the type of foods that you consume, you should certainly up your protein consumption, while you must also remember that every meal should be as well balanced as possible. Nevertheless, protein is the bedrock on which muscle is built, so a significant percentage of the additional calories that you are ingesting should be in the form of proteins.

Next, you should commence a solid program of weight training if you have not already done so, because it is by weight training that you stimulate your muscles to grow, and it is the growth of your muscles that channels most of the additional energy that you are taking in every day in that direction (as opposed to building fat stores).

However, it is inevitable that while you are trying to channel most of the surplus energy in the direction of building additional muscle mass, a certain percentage of it will accumulate as body fat.

The final phase of your body building efforts once the muscle mass is increasing is to encourage your body to do exactly what it doesn't want to do, which is to become catabolic and anabolic at the same time.

While this is not going to happen overnight, after some weeks or months of weight training and eating to build muscle mass, you should see that your physique and basic shape has already changed significantly. In short, you will have added muscle mass, but you will also have added some extra fat.

However, this is not the same as some overweight or obese individual who could serve as a poster boy (or girl) for couch potatoes everywhere! In other words, while you will have put on a little more fat, you will still nevertheless be possessed of far more muscle mass than you were previously, so your need to lose weight is entirely different from that of the average obese person.

Nevertheless, if you want to shed the final few pounds of fat so that you achieve the classic bodybuilder physique, you do need to convince your body to do what it does not want to do. This is a strategy that all professional or high-level competition bodybuilders have to go through on a regular basis, a process that is known as 'cutting', the removal of the final few pounds of excess fat that allows the muscle mass to shine through.

To do this, your diet has to be extremely low in fat (less than 20%) while maintaining a high level of protein to protect and promote the muscle mass which you have been working on with such dedication. Keep protein intake at least as high as in previous weeks and months, while cutting down on sugars, sweets and white flour products and maintaining your intake of antioxidant fresh fruits and vegetables.

Taking the two diet phases step-by-step, you might therefore end up with a bodybuilding diet that looks something like this:

Phase 1 – 'Building mass' or bulking phase

Carbohydrates: 50% to 60%

Proteins: 15% to 20%

Fats: 20% to 30%

Phase 2 – Trimming down or cutting phase

Carbohydrates: 50% to 60%

Proteins: 20% to 30%

Fats: 10% to 20%

One note of caution that you should heed is that these numbers, particularly the intake of proteins, are at the top end of the acceptable scale, so do keep an eye on your general health. Although overconsumption of proteins is not likely to harm any healthy, fit individual, you should nevertheless exercise care. For example, if there is any indication of kidney problems, you should consult a medical professional immediately.

The American College of Sports Medicine suggests that the ideal protein consumption for a top-level athlete who is constantly training is in the region of 1.6 to 1.7 g of protein materials per kilogram of body weight, so bear this number in mind when you are calculating the amount of proteins that you are consuming either while bulking up, or (more importantly) when you are trying to trim down.

If at all possible, take these proteins as part of your normal daily diet, rather than ingesting a huge number of protein shakes and the like every day.

While if you are using some kind of trainer to help you build the physique you are looking for, you may find that they are very heavily in favor of using supplements of this nature, it is far better if you can eat the proteins that you need as a part of your normal daily diet.

If there is no other reason for this, buying huge amounts of protein shakes can become extremely expensive, which might take some of the fun out of what you are doing if your body building efforts are for your own satisfaction only!

Should You Supplement with Natural Protein?

Discussion of body building supplements always creates a lot of controversy. Of course, some are illegal, some are ineffective and some are downright dangerous. The one body building supplement that you can't go wrong with is natural protein. Not only is protein

There is one particular body building supplement that after time and time again has been proven to be one of the best supplements any body builder could use. This particular body building supplement, that can also be found naturally, is protein.

The muscle needs the protein in order to grow. When a body builder or any person getting fit lifts weights, the intake of protein then has a stimulating effect on the muscle tissue and acts as the best muscle enhancement supplement that the body could offer. In terms of saving muscle, if one does a massive amount of cardio (either high intensity or low intensity for an extended period of time) the body will burn all its carb stores and then will start burning muscle.

Then when your body starts to use up its carbs that are stored it will not automatically just burn fat, it will also start to burn muscle. The protein body building supplement will then help the body replace any muscle burned away from an intensive workout.

Protein can be found naturally in chicken and other meat sources, but the worry is that a massive amount of protein would have to be digested to be helpful, therefore a body builder would have to eat much meat. A protein body building supplement could help with the natural intake of protein.

Be careful when using the protein shakes that are loaded with sugar. Sugar will make you fat quickly, so stick with the low sugar content protein body building supplements. Usually, the high sugar protein powders are the flavors that are too good to be true such as "Chocolate Chip Cookie Dough" or "Blueberry Cheesecake." Avoid this and stick with something more realistic like banana flavored or vanilla flavored, as less sugar will be in these particular flavors. There is also unflavored protein shake powder as well. Whatever supplement you decide to choose, remember to choose your supplement carefully.

Chapter 10 – Does the Acai Berry Diet Really Work?

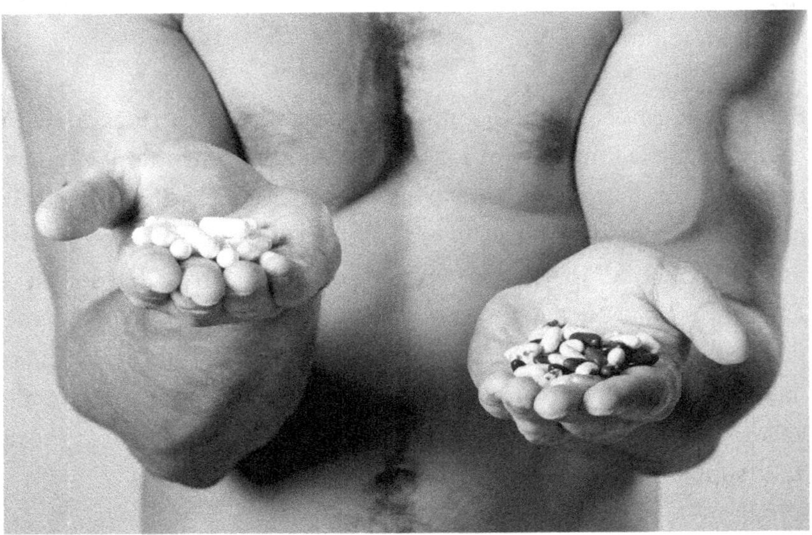

Many Muscle building diets are built on whole foods where carbs and other essential nutrient components are drawn from. Muscle builders have to refrain from getting nutrients from processed foods. The acai berry is one of the remarkable protein sources in healthy eating circles. The fruit has numerous benefits for weight loss and body building and thus is a suggested alternative in muscle building diets. There is much that has been published about the power acai berries especially on the aspects of weight-loss and eye sight, cardiovascular, etc. Not much though has been published on the benefits of the acai berry on muscle building.

Muscles are built out of proteins. This is the reason why many body building diets are made of foods which are rich in protein. Proteins do not get to the body as hard protein directly but they get to the body as amino acids. The amino acids are like the building blocks for the proteins. The acai berry is rich in amino acids and will verily boost the levels of proteins in your body. You need not to rely on these only but have to make use of them in tandem with a holistic diet which will ensure that your energy and nutritive requirements are in synch with your fitness goals.

What you need to know is that there are over 7 types of amino acids in the acai berry. The proportion of the amino acids in the acai berry supplement is a very significant proportion in comparisons to other foods. You can get acai berries through various products which enlist pulps and juices as well as powders. As a body builder you have to lay your hands on these products and make sure that you have a protein rich diet to match the energy and nutritive demands of your active body. Acai berries are also rich in antioxidants and remove bad cholesterol from the body. The antioxidants are effective in helping the body's digestive system and all other metabolism related functionalities. The acai berries are specifically known to be effective in getting rid of the harmful LDL cholesterol. The effects of acai berries result in a trimmed body which will be quite easy to work with as you pace towards your health and fitness goals

- The health benefits of Acai Berries

Acai berry supplements have become one of the most remarkable alternatives and breakthroughs in the health and nutrition industry. Acai Berry is the buzz phrase in today's health and nutrition circles and its supplements are topping the shopping priorities for health conscious consumers. Acai berries are rich in antioxidants which are the reason why the berries and supplement alternatives have topped lists in weight-loss and healthy living diets and menus. Acai berries are picked from unique palm trees that are found in the Amazon. The berries come with loads of health benefits like the reduction of chances of developing cancer, keeping the heart healthy and protecting from Alzheimer form of diseases.

- Acai berries are good for rest

Acai berry supplements are effective in enhancing the effectiveness of your body systems and helping you to rest in a rejuvenating way. Acai berries are commended for their components which promote restful sleep which is an important ingredient of a stress free lifestyle. Acai berries products and supplements are good for people who find it hard to sleep and are persistently restless. Acai berries have proved to be good remedy for fatigue related problems. Upon enhancing your restfulness and refreshing your body acai berries come with energy boosting components. The good aspect about the acai berry supplements is that they are natural unlike other stimulants and caffeine products which come with side effects.

- Preparation of Acai berries

What makes acai berry supplements a good alternative is the manner in which the harvested berries are prepared. Acai supplements are healthier since the production process of the berries is largely through the freeze drying method which ensures that the vital nutrition components of the berries are retained. Berries used for acai supplements are subjected to freeze drying just after they are gathered and this method has made acai supplements more superior than other so called energy products made of fruits processed through methods such as drum drying. Acai berries supplements are replete with the vital energy giving components which are retained through the delicate freeze drying methods.

- Merits of acai berry supplements

Owing to the natural nutrition components of the acai berry supplements and the way in which the berries are prepared through the freeze dry methods acai berry supplements are an easy choice for health conscious buyers. The acai supplements have a high energy value and nutrition components which are essential for healthy living. Bodies fed with acai berry supplement are in a better condition to resist diseases and enhance the immunity system as well as improve the digestive system. Research has also indicated that health components found in acai berries are essential for diminishing the effects of ageing as well as enhancing vision. The crucial merit of the acai berry supplements is that they come with a holistic set of vital natural component which revive the body and keep the body in a good condition to fight and resist disease.

CHAPTER 11 – THE BODY BUILDER'S LIFESTYLE

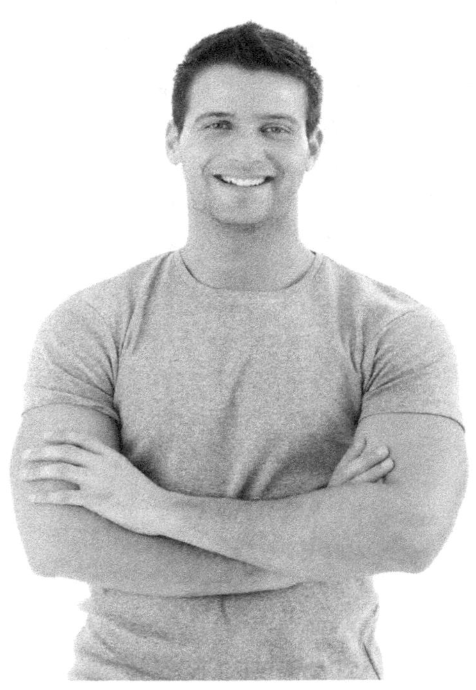

To a degree, everything you do in your efforts to increase muscle mass is a lifestyle decision. However, in this section of the report, I am not going to refer to the hours that you have to find to be able to train in order to become a bodybuilder or even the lifestyle impacts of changing your diet to one that is more conducive to building muscle mass.

Instead, this section of the report will focus on other aspects of your life where you can make changes that will help you to become a better, more successful bodybuilder completely naturally.

The primary objective of anyone who is attempting to become a successful bodybuilder is to develop existing muscles by adding mass while also reducing the percentage of body fat you carry around with you. Anything that acts in the opposite manner to either of these pre-requisites is going to damage your attempts to be a serious natural bodybuilder.

How Stress Affects Your Bodybuilding Efforts

Cortisol is a hormone that is produced by the adrenal cortex, which is part of the adrenal gland. It is a hormone that is often referred to as the 'stress' hormone which increases both blood sugar levels and pressure, while also reducing the effectiveness of your immune system.

Perhaps the most important thing about cortisol is that it has been indicated that when it is produced in excess amounts (i.e. in response to increased stress or tension levels), it can reduce muscle mass while aiding the deposit of additional body fat.

From this observation, it naturally follows that if you are trying to become a more successful bodybuilder, you need to reduce cortisol levels if at all possible.

The first thing that you can do in an attempt to reduce cortisol is to reduce the stress that is present in your everyday life.

For example, try to teach yourself time management skills and how to keep every day, whether working or at leisure, completely under control.

Instead of leaving everything to the last minute so it becomes a panic filled rush, plan everything you do every day well ahead of time. In addition, give yourself plenty of time to make sure that you achieve everything you want to achieve, because there is nothing more likely to cause stress and tension than either having to leave a job uncompleted or having to finish it in a mad rush in order to get everything done.

Consider learning additional skills that will help to keep your stress levels under control such as yoga, meditation and how to breathe properly, as an aid to keeping self-control. All of these practices will greatly assist you in reducing the stress levels that you currently feel every day and as a result, the level of cortisol circulating in your body will naturally decrease.

Another thing that can help to reduce stress and therefore the levels of cortisol that your adrenal cortex is producing is to make sure that you get enough sleep. Most experts recommend that a healthy, restorative good night's sleep is made up of 8 hours and 15 minutes of solid rest.

However, while you are trying to reduce the stress levels in your life, it is often not possible to make everything perfect, simply because there are not enough hours in the day for each of us to pack in everything that we want to do. Hence, if 8 hours and 15 minutes of sound sleep is not possible, you should aim for at least 7 hours of total rest every night, and make up the rest either with a late afternoon nap or at the weekend.

This is important, because it is scientifically proven that a lack of sleep greatly increases the production of cortisol, which will significantly hinder the effectiveness of your bodybuilding efforts and add fat to your torso at the same time.

Happiness and balance is an important factor in your bodybuilding success as well. This is because bodybuilding is a 24 hour activity, something that you cannot pick up and put down as you see fit. It requires a certain degree of dedication and a lot of determination, but living a balanced life is important too because doing things away from the gym that you enjoy doing makes it easier to put up with the training when it is hard.

Removing Harmful Habits

While your efforts to become a successful natural bodybuilder will necessitate following a program of training that is specifically designed to build muscle mass, it is important to appreciate that living a generally healthy lifestyle is a central part of achieving balance and happiness as well.

So, while weights and the like are an essential part of your bodybuilding efforts, lifting weights is an anaerobic sport, an activity that does not give your heart and lungs a workout.

Consequently, you should also consider practicing aerobic sports like swimming or cycling, and if you can find something that you really enjoy doing at the same time, so much the better. Taking up something like swimming will greatly increase your endurance and stamina, and if you enjoy it as well, it inevitably makes the necessary hard work in the gym seem that much easier to bear.

The bottom line is that becoming a successful natural bodybuilder is not something that is going to happen overnight, and there will be times when your progress might seem slower than you would like it to be.

It is at times like these, when having other things in your life, things that you can turn to for enjoyment that are nevertheless good for you, will sometimes be the escape valve that you need. Without this escape valve, you come back to the fact that you will be stressed, you will be tense and you already know how this can adversely affect your efforts.

Building a Bigger, Leaner Body

This is not to suggest that everything you do should relate to exercise. Indeed, your life should definitely not only be focused on exercise, because rest is an essential part of being a successful bodybuilder.

There is also a school of thought that maintains that too much aerobic or cardiovascular exercise can increase the production of cortisol, so it is essential that you keep your cardiovascular exercise in the 'fat burning zone'.

This is one reason why, for a non-competitive bodybuilder, the best time to undertake aerobic exercise is immediately after a weights session.

By doing so, you ensure that the excess glycogen in your body (the first source of energy that your body turns to before it starts to burn the fat) has been exhausted by your weight training before you start exercising. Therefore, as soon as you start aerobic exercise, you are straight into the 'fat burning zone' the minute you start.

Remembering that there is a counterbalance between the importance of burning fat and accumulating muscle mass, this ability to start burning fat immediately after a weights session is an excellent way of keeping your body fat percentage to a minimum.

As an approximate formula by which you calculate the point at which you enter the 'fat burning zone', use this formula:

$$FBZ = 220 - (\text{your age}) \times 0.75$$

This will give you an approximate idea of how many heartbeats a minute you need to experience in order to start burning fat. Once you are in this 'zone', the average male should aim for 5 or 6 aerobic exercise sessions a week for 30 minutes a time, whereas females should be looking at 20-30 minutes the same number of times every week. Stick to these limits, and the risk of getting into a situation where you amplify cortisol production is very limited.

There must be times when you get away from all forms of training and exercise to make an effort to relax. But when you do so, try not to succumb to bad practices that might actually damage your bodybuilding efforts.

For example, while having the occasional beer is not going to damage the chances of your being a successful bodybuilder very much, smoking 20 cigarettes a day is certainly going to make it an awful lot harder to achieve the physique that you want to achieve.

Filling your lungs with tar and nicotine filled smoke every day is likely to reduce your ability to recover from serious training sessions, meaning that you will automatically be able to train less frequently and probably with less intensity as well. Your progress to bodybuilding success will naturally be slowed if you are a heavy smoker.

One of the greatest personal characteristics that you will learn or have enhanced by becoming a natural bodybuilder is that of personal discipline, which is a prerequisite for taking a life changing decision like quitting the evil weed!

Remember to apply determination and discipline to everything in your life, and set goals in everything you do as a way of achieving and then maintaining the balance that you must have to be successful.

Getting the body that you want is going to take a lot of hard work and effort, so only a naïve fool would believe that it's going to be easy to achieve your goals. However, once you do get to where you want to be in bodybuilding terms, you can live what you might call the 'bodybuilder lifestyle' in the same way as thousands of other successful bodybuilders.

Nevertheless, do not ever allow yourself to lose sight of the fact that the lifestyle is not your whole life. You need balance, you need outside interests away from the gym, and above all else, you have to adapt an all-round lifestyle that is conducive to achieving bodybuilding success.

CHAPTER 12 – PREVENTING COMMON BODY BUILDING INJURIES

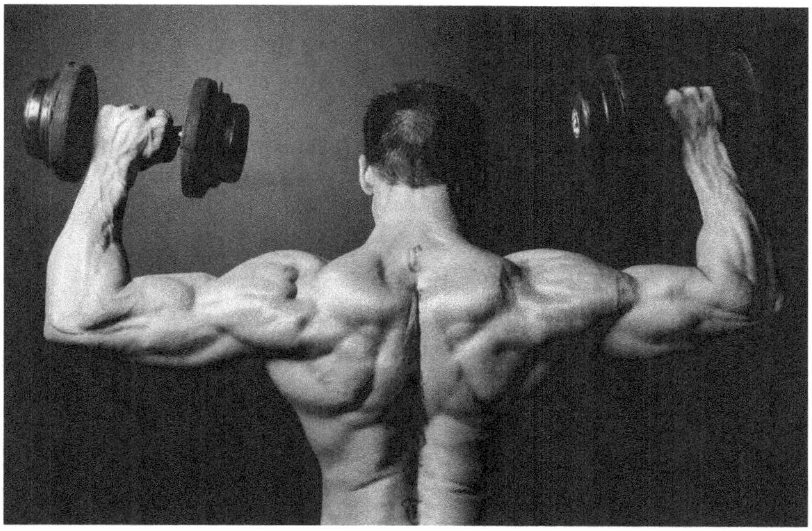

As careful as we are in life, we all tend to incur certain injuries from time to time. Bodybuilders are probably more susceptible to these injuries, especially beginners eager to get in a forceful workout. Most bodybuilding injuries occur from not having a proper workout before starting your routines or improperly using the body. Here are just a few of the most common injuries and ways you can prevent them.

Abdominal strain occurs when your abdominal muscles are strained during a forceful activity such as lifting a heavy object without proper warm-ups. Symptoms may be inflammation or tenderness at the bottom of your abdomen, a sharp in abdominal muscles or when contracting these muscles. Abdominal strain can be prevented by making sure your abdomen is well toned before working out. Crunches, sit ups, running or using stationary bikes and treadmills are great ways to warm up before you begin your routines.

Calf strain is very common with beginner bodybuilders and occurs when the tendons and muscles in the lower back part of your leg incur an injury, most often from forcefully pushing off your toes such as with jumping, running or lunging. Difficulty in standing on your tiptoes or contracting your knee, swelling and pain in the calf muscle and sudden pain in the lower back leg are all symptoms of calf strain. Prevention of calf strain takes place by doing proper warm ups like sit ups, running or working out on an exercise bike, treadmill, stepper or with dumbbells.

Lower back pain is probably one of the most painful injuries and occurs when a muscle or ligament that's near a vertebra is strained. Because your nerves go to all parts of your body, lower back pain can cause weakness or pain anywhere in your body. Symptoms are possible bruising or swelling in a ruptured area, sudden pain in your back and difficulty in moving. Lower back pain can be preventing by using your legs rather than your arms and back to lift heavy objects, sitting in a straight backed chair and avoiding lifting more than you can comfortably carry.

Achilles tendonitis is when your Achilles tendon is inflamed and causes pain on the back part of your leg near your heel. It can occur when the Achilles tendon is overused, from consistent uphill running or from increased sports or strength training. Achilles tendonitis can be prevented by stretching your Achilles tendons and calf muscles before you begin your workout. If you notice that you have a tendency to have Achilles problems, avoid any uphill running.

In the case of any injury, do not apply any heat, drink alcohol or have a massage within 24 hours of the injury. For the best recovery of most injuries, apply the RICE treatment, which includes Rest, Ice, Compression and Elevation.

CHAPTER 13 – CHOOSING THE BEST TRAINER FOR YOU

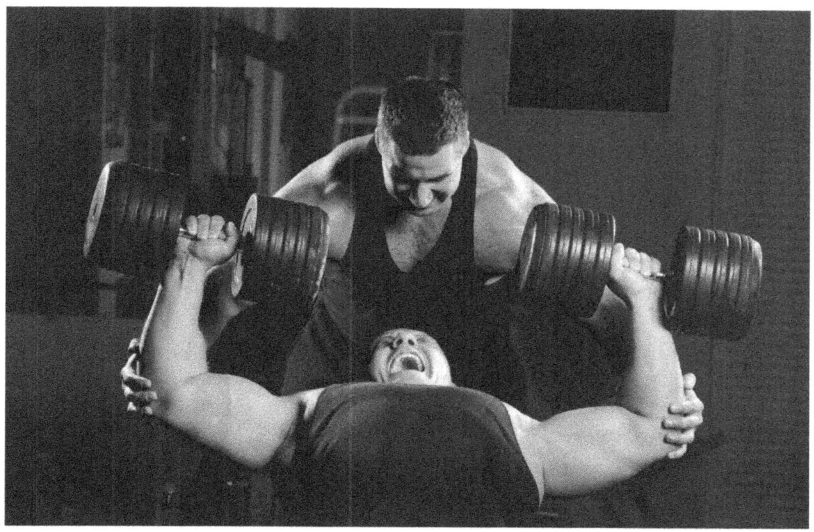

You've finally made the decision to get into bodybuilding, which has been your dream for a long time. You want to be successful at bodybuilding so you can be healthier and have a body you can be proud of. All your research has indicated that, for your best chance at success, you should hire a professional bodybuilding trainer.

Do you know what to look for in a professional bodybuilding trainer? Here are some simple tips on what you should look for in a professional bodybuilding trainer or some of the required qualifications.

• Any trainer you're even considering should care about your goals, expectations and limitations. The trainer should take the time to get to know you and your personality. He or she should also get to know about what exercises or foods you enjoy and what your overall goals may be so he can implement a bodybuilding program that meets your needs and fits into your lifestyle.

Programs should not be one size fits all but rather designed for each individual.

- A qualified trainer will always care about your health first and will want to get clearance from your doctor. The trainer should not just take your word for it that you're healthy. To maintain your good health and protect his or her legal liability, the trainer should not begin working with you until clearance has been given.

- The trainer should be the type of person that will keep you motivated and make you feel comfortable working with them. They should not be bossy or intimidating in any way. Keep in mind that you'll be working together a lot so you want a trainer that you're comfortable around. If you have any questions, you'll want someone with a personable attitude and someone that has the patience to answer your questions and address your concerns.

- Your trainer should pay attention to your progress and how you're doing overall. Being your trainer involves more than just being paid from you. The trainer should care about their client and want to see them succeed at their goals. A good trainer is going to be well educated on nutritional needs and any questions you may have about diets, supplements, etc. Any trainer that's good at the job will always set a good example for you in exercise and diet.

- Don't be afraid to ask for references. If this is a good trainer, he will not only provide you with references but will encourage you to check with other clients. Speak with the references and ask them how they felt about this person as a trainer and get as much information as possible.

Keys to a Successful Bodybuilding Session

Bodybuilding takes place in many sizes, shapes and forms so to speak. The type of bodybuilding technique you use will depend a lot on the part of your body you're focusing on the most. While some bodybuilders focus on just one or two parts of their body, others will work on the entire body.

The intensity of your workout is very important for your success. In fact, many professional trainers believe it's every bit as important as the exercises you're doing. Here are a few tips on how to make your workouts count the most.

Make your workouts short. A workout that lasts an hour is perfect, although it can vary from 45 to 75 minutes. Your body produces certain fat burning and muscle building hormones, which help with your bodybuilding. However, after 75 minutes the levels of these hormones begin to drop, which will not only not help you anymore, but also can actually slow down your process. More is not always better, especially with bodybuilding.

Take short breaks in between each different set. A minute and a half is the longest your rest should be so you can still meet your goals while not going longer than 75 minutes. Research shows that this type of training will not only stimulate your hormone growth but will also do wonders for your cardiovascular system.

Each exercise set should consist of 8 to 15 repetitions for the best increase in muscle mass. By keeping the repetitions in this range, you're getting the best blood flow to your muscle cells. Along with blood flow, you are also providing your muscles mass with needed nutrients. Studies have shown that the most productive fat burning and muscle building occurs at this range of repetitions.

Stay with weights you can control. Another bonus of doing this many repetitions is that logic says if you're doing this many, you're using a weight that you can comfortably control. Too many people make the mistake of starting with weights they cannot control, believing they'll develop muscle mass much quicker. They just become sore and tired quicker!

Add variety to your sessions. Every bodybuilder has a favorite exercise and wants to do that all the time. However, the best way to continually grow your muscles is with variety. You'll also find you're more motivated and enthusiastic when you're trying a new variety of bodybuilding exercise. As you get more familiar and experienced with your bodybuilding routine, you'll find that you'll want to get into more repetitions and more different sessions, while still keeping each one within the required 75 minute period.

CHAPTER 14 – BODY BUILDING FOR THE LADIES

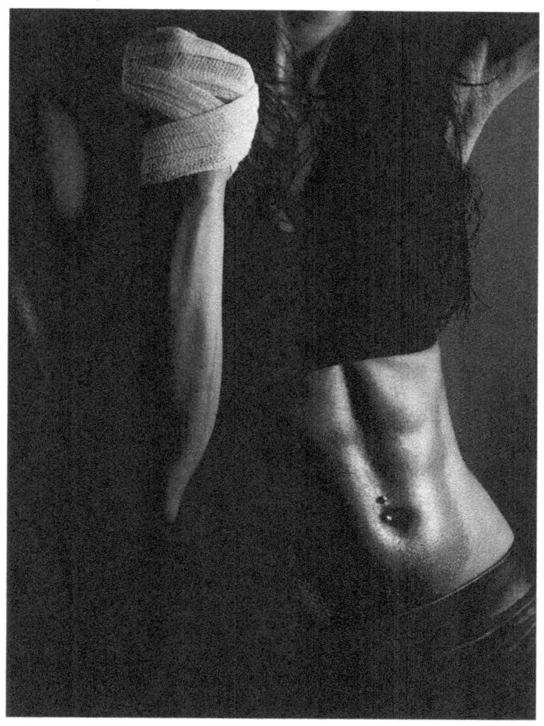

Bodybuilding has really increased in popularity in recent years. Female bodybuilding has also gained popularity in huge numbers. With the emphasis the world in making on physical fitness and its importance for overall good health, women are turning to bodybuilding. Female bodybuilding is to not only help develop curves in the right places but also to develop and keep their muscles toned and firm. Proper bodybuilding workouts can help to form the muscles and shape up a woman's body as well as improve their physical strength and promote good health.

Difference in the Genders

Female bodybuilding is not very different from male bodybuilding. After all, men and women both have the same number of muscles in their bodies. They also appear to get the same results from a physical workout. There is one major difference between men and women, at least one in regards to bodybuilding. Men have testosterone, which is a hormone that helps to build muscles while women have estrogen, which is a hormone known for storing fat. This does not mean that women will gain weight quicker than men will, however. A female that's working out can easily build muscles and lose fat.

Misconceptions on Female Bodybuilding

Many women would love to have a strong and muscular body, but are afraid to participate in bodybuilding because they fear that if they quit, their newly developed muscles will instantly turn to fat. This is virtually impossible in spite of how widely believed it's been. Muscle and fat are two very different tissues. Fat develops when the body stores unburned calories because these calories have not been burned because of a decrease of physical activity. This will happen to any individual that is suddenly inactive, including bodybuilders. Muscles will never turn into fat.

Benefits of Female Bodybuilding

There are many benefits to female bodybuilding. While many women are afraid they will suddenly develop a bulky muscular body and lose their femininity, this is not the case. When bodybuilding is properly done with consistency, they can develop a curvaceous body that looks years longer than it actually is. Bodybuilding routines for the arms, for instance, can help eliminate the weak and flabby upper arms that often develop with age. This is just one example of what female bodybuilding can achieve.

Because women's bodies are made differently than men, the weight training requirements for women are going to be different as well. It's not going to be quite as easy for a woman to bulk up from bodybuilding. Female bodybuilding requires exercises will also target your cardiovascular system, which will give your body a much needed health bonus. Let's face the fact that all woman want to have the perfect body and have it for as long as possible. With the right kind of systemic weight training, this can be possible.

ABOUT THE AUTHOR

Andrew Jackson is a professional body builder and a chiropractor. He has won national body building competitions and is often referred to as the ideal man.

Andrew was born on June 4, 1980. He was the third in a brood of 5. His parents, Jenny and Perry, were high school sweethearts. They were raised in love.